JUAN CARLOS CORAL

Cancer's Echo: Why Me?

From Fear to Faith: A Survivor's Tale of Triumph and Healing. Overcoming Cancer with Determination, Medical Treatment, Nutrition, Spirit, and the Power of Love.

First edition

This book was professionally typeset on Reedsy.
Find out more at reedsy.com

Contents

1

Introduction

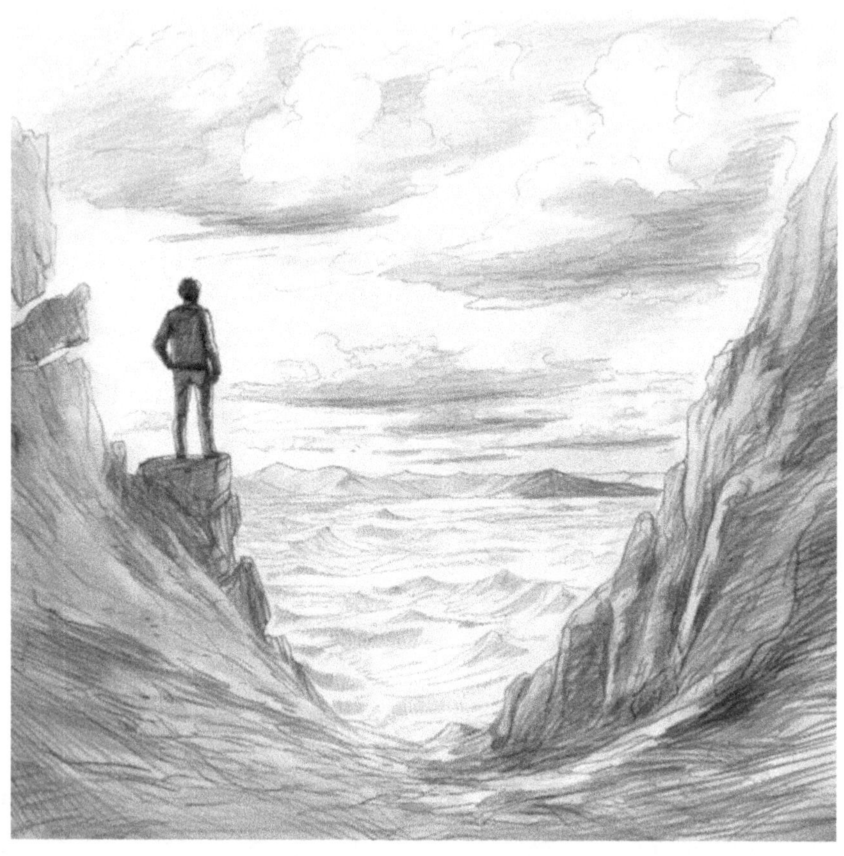

From the moment life thrusts an unexpected blow, we are faced with the profound decision to sink or to soar. In a fleeting instant, nestled between a doctor's concerned gaze and the deafening silence that follows life-altering news, I found myself grappling with a question that became the title of this journey: *"Cancer... Why me?"* I am no different from you; I once moved through life with routine normalcy, valuing moments but perhaps taking many for granted. But there's an inexplicable transformation that occurs when life's fragility becomes palpably clear. My story, like many others, began on an ordinary day, when the future was a series of aspirations, dreams, and daily routines. However, on a day I least expected, the universe presented a challenge, enveloped in a word we all fear: "*Cancer.*" It prompts us to evaluate everything — our purpose, our connections, our very essence.

This book is an open door into the intimate corners of my soul, the whispered prayers during sleepless nights, the moments of raw vulnerability, and the indefatigable strength found in the embrace of loved ones. It's a testament to the boundless human spirit that seeks to thrive even when the odds are stacked against it. My intent is not just to share a story, but to offer you a lantern in what may seem like an insurmountable darkness. Within these pages you find a testament of faith, the transformative power of love, and the age-old belief that the mind, when harnessed, has the power to heal, renew, and rejuvenate.

You'll journey with me from the days of blissful ignorance, through the crushing weight of diagnosis, to the arduous path of healing and eventual victory. But more than that, this book seeks to be a beacon for those who ask the questions we all, at some point, whisper to the universe: "*Why me? Why this? Why now?*" By the end of our journey together, it is my sincerest hope that you will have found your answers or at least embarked on your own quest of understanding and resilience.

This isn't just a recount of medical procedures and healing regimens; it's a story about rediscovering oneself amidst chaos, about the delicate balance of surrendering and fighting, and about realizing that in our most vulnerable moments, we often find our mightiest strengths.

Why share this journey? Because stories have an innate power. They transcend time, resonate with the soul, and remind us that we are not alone in our battles. As you turn each page, I hope you find fragments of your own strength, reflections of your own love, and the silent echo of your own heartbeat, urging you to believe, to hope, and to persevere.

Now, let's go back to where it all began, to the day life paused, rewound, and played a track I was neither expecting nor prepared for. Walk with me to the genesis of this tale, when I first heard the words that changed everything. Let's dive into 'The News'.

2

The News

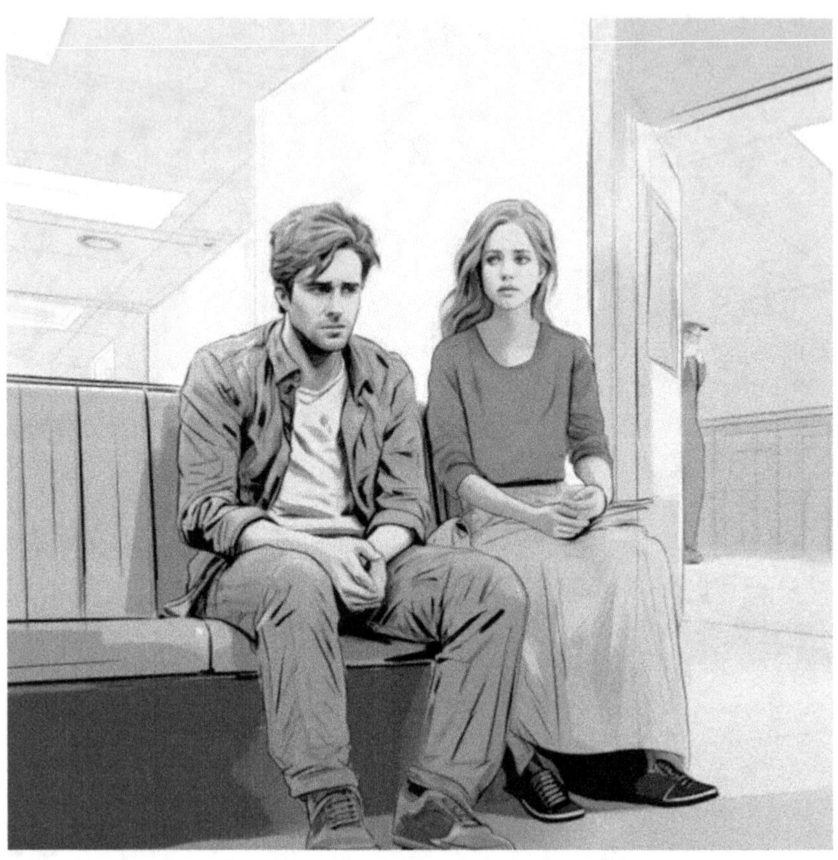

L ife is often likened to a journey, a series of twists and turns with unexpected detours that challenge our resilience and determination. Most days, the path is predictable, marked by routine, familiarity, and the comfort of the known. But every so often, we encounter a fork in the road that stops us in our tracks, forcing us to re-calibrate our direction and purpose. It's in these defining moments that our character is truly tested, where our deepest fears meet our strongest resolve. As I sat in that cold waiting room, awaiting the news that would forever alter my path, I was on the cusp of one such defining moment.

The Monster in the Waiting Room

There's a certain level of detachment we all maintain from life's tragedies. The stories we hear on the news, the tales of others, always feel like they're happening in some distant world, far removed from our daily reality. Until the day when it crashes into your life, and suddenly that protective bubble you lived in bursts wide open.

Every so often, life presents us with moments that feel so surreal, they're almost like scenes from a movie—only, there's no director yelling "*cut.*" I was in such a moment.

The cold, sterile environment of the hospital seemed to magnify the heaviness in the air. The hum of fluorescent lights overhead was almost rhythmic, and the muted conversations in the distance were punctuated by the occasional cough or shuffle of feet. But all of that faded to mere background noise as I waited, a lingering dizziness from anesthesia clouding the edges of my perception.

Then, cutting through the haze, came the doctor's voice. His words felt like they were delivered from miles away, and yet, they bore down on me with an immediate and crushing weight. Tumors. Colon. Life expectancy. The syllables hung in the air like a death knell, shattering the cocoon of denial I had wrapped myself in. Those words felt disjointed, yet together they formed a dark cloud that threatened the very fabric of my existence. Suddenly, the myriad of dreams, plans, and moments I'd taken for granted seemed to be snatched away, replaced by this monstrous reality. It was as if a monster had entered the waiting room, lurking in the corners, waiting to devour all the hopes and dreams I'd so carefully nurtured.

Why Me?

In the aftermath of those words, there was a silence. A stillness that seemed to stretch on for an eternity. I saw my life, not as a continuous journey but as a series of vivid snapshots – the joy of childhood, the thrill of young love, the pride of parenthood. Thoughts flashed in rapid succession. The dreams I held onto of watching my children grow, of growing old beside my wife, and of completing those projects that were mere sketches in my mind. They all seemed so far away, so unattainable now.

A chilling fear crept over me, rooted in memories of my father. His own battle with cancer had been a shadow over our family, a haunting reminder of the fragility of life. His journey, filled with pain, resilience, and eventually, loss, was a story I'd hoped would remain as a tale of the past. But now, the specter of that disease threatened to consume my own narrative. It's a sobering realization when you understand that cancer, an adversary we often associate with others, was now a part of my story too. Virtually everyone knows someone who's battled with cancer, but nothing truly prepares you for the day it becomes personal.

The weight of realization settled in: these tragedies weren't exclusive to "*others*." I wasn't exempt from the cruel twists of fate. The enormity of it all bore down on me, pressing against my chest, making each breath feel labored. The world seemed to blur around me, and in its center, was this profound sense of injustice. It's an indescribable feeling when the adversities we've only heard about, believing they belong to others, suddenly claim a space in our own story. The safety and predictability of life, as I knew it, crumbled. A singular question raced through my mind, echoing off the walls of my consciousness, desperate for an answer: "*Why is this happening to me?*"

It was a plea to the universe, to life, and to God. A question born from a mix of shock, disbelief, and an overwhelming sense of vulnerability. But in that moment, amidst the turmoil and despair, there also emerged a spark – a determination to seek answers, to understand, and to fight against the monster that had dared to enter my world.

3

How Did Life Used to Be?

Life, as I knew it, was a canvas of colors, each hue representing the myriad tasks, responsibilities, and activities that filled my days. Each morning brought its own rhythm—a blare of alarm clocks, the aroma of brewing coffee, music on the radio, and the routine of checking on the day's agenda. The hours would be crammed with deadlines and meetings, interspersed with laughter and conversations over lunch breaks, and punctuated by the humdrum of daily commutes.

In today's world, many of us have unknowingly become slaves to the very technology designed to simplify our lives. Endless scrolling through social media feeds, habitually checking emails outside of work hours, binge-watching the latest trending shows, or getting lost in the vortex of online shopping—all these activities, while seemingly innocuous, consumed chunks of our precious time. What was once a tool for connection turned into hours of comparison, lost amidst the curated highlights of others' lives.

Furthermore, the pursuit of a perfect world added its own layer of stress. A world where we're constantly bombarded with ideals—perfect homes straight out of a magazine, exotic holidays flaunted on social media, or the incessant chase for the latest gadgets. The pressure to keep up, to mold our lives according to these constructed ideals, led to an ongoing cycle of work and spend, often sidelining what truly mattered.

Amid this whirlwind of activities and distractions, genuine moments of connection—deep conversations, nature walks, reading a book, or even just sitting in reflective silence—became rarer. Many found themselves overbooked yet under connected, busy yet unfulfilled.

We became experts at '*being busy*', priding ourselves on juggling multiple roles and responsibilities, all the while neglecting the very core of our existence—our well-being, our passions, our relationships, and the pursuit of genuine happiness.

I, too, was caught up in this whirlwind. The weight of pursuing an "*ideal life*" persisted. Complaints were frequent—about the traffic, the workload, the fleeting weekends—and each problem felt monumental, until the next one came along, dwarfing its predecessor.

Isn't it strange how we give undue importance to trivialities, elevating minor inconveniences to monumental challenges? We often lament about the inconsequential, allowing it to consume our thoughts and energy, only to realize its insignificance when faced with a true crisis.

And then, the diagnosis. Cancer. A word that instantly eclipsed every other concern, casting them into irrelevance. All the previous complaints, worries, and stresses that seemed so paramount suddenly faded into obscurity. The gravity of this new challenge dwarfed everything else. It was a stark reminder of the fragility and unpredictability of life. In the face of genuine adversity, it became painfully clear how much time and energy had been wasted on the inconsequential.

4

Back to the Harsh Reality

L ife has an uncanny way of blindsiding us. Just when we think we've charted our course, understood our rhythm, and settled into our groove, it throws us a curveball. For many, these unexpected turns are mere blips on the radar, manageable disruptions that are navigated with grace. But there are some turns so sharp, so earth-shattering, that they redefine the very essence of our existence. My diagnosis was one such pivotal moment—a dramatic pause, a deep breath, a re-calibration of everything I thought I knew.

How Bad Is This?

Nightmares have a peculiar trait; they terrify, but when you jolt awake, the palpable relief that follows is almost cathartic. The shadows fade, the heart rate slows, and the world regains its clarity. But what if the nightmare doesn't end when you open your eyes? That was the sensation that gripped me. Each morning, in the quiet solitude of dawn, I would find a fleeting moment of forgetfulness, only for the weight of reality to crash upon me. The word 'cancer' hung in the air, a persistent cloud casting a shadow over each waking moment. Information came in torrents—medical jargon, statistics, treatment options. The enormity of what lay ahead was both overwhelming and suffocating.

Upon hearing the term '*cancer*', a myriad of thoughts raced through my mind. Cancer isn't just one disease; it's a spectrum of disorders with varying degrees of aggression, potential for spread, and prognosis. There's the earliest stage where it's localized, offering a glimmer of hope for a complete cure. Then, there are more advanced stages, where the disease has spread, making treatment more complex. There's also the aggressive nature of certain types, and the more indolent, slow-growing others. The trepidation stemmed from not knowing where I fit within this spectrum.

While I awaited further details, the anguish of uncertainty weighed heavily. Would I be dealing with a treatable, early-stage cancer that required minimal intervention? Or was I about to embark on a grueling journey through the rigorous world of chemotherapy, radiation, and surgeries? The difference in outcomes between these scenarios was vast. One hinted at a relatively swift return to normalcy, while the other promised months, if not years, of physical and emotional battles.

The Options I Have

Reactions to life-altering news vary vastly. Some rage against the unfairness of it all, others bury their heads in the sand, hoping that avoidance might somehow alter reality. Denial, anger, fear, bargaining— emotions ebb and flow like tidal waves, each trying to make sense of the inexplicable. But amidst this tempest of feelings, a realization struck with crystal clarity: the path forward was singular.

In the vast expanse of life's challenges, every cloud, no matter how dark, possesses a silver lining. And even in the face of something as daunting as cancer, choices present themselves, offering pathways that can lead to healing, growth, and transformation. The more I dove into understanding my situation, the more it became clear that I was far from powerless.

While the initial shock might have painted a picture of limited choices, the reality was different. Medical advancements have brought forth a plethora of treatment options tailored to specific cancer types and stages. From minimally invasive surgeries to targeted therapies that home in on the very cells causing the illness, modern medicine has given patients a fighting chance like never before. And beyond the conventional, there are holistic approaches, focusing on nutrition, mental well-being, and alternative therapies that complement traditional treatments and enhance recovery.

Beyond the medical realm, the choices extended to my mindset and approach. I could choose to view this diagnosis as a death sentence, or I could see it as a life lesson. A call to truly value each day, to deepen connections with loved ones, and to discover reservoirs of strength I never knew I had. This was an opportunity, albeit a tough one, to reevaluate, re-calibrate, and emerge even stronger. Armed with knowledge, surrounded by support, and fueled by a spirit of resilience, the options before me were clear. I could, and would, embark on this journey with hope, determination, and a conviction to not just survive but to truly thrive.

Surrender wasn't an option; neither was self-pity. While the journey ahead was fraught with uncertainty, the decision was firm. It was time to gear up for the fight, to face this adversary head-on.

Ok...So, What's Next?

Committing to the battle is one thing, navigating its intricacies is another. Cancer isn't just a disease; it's a maze of tests, treatments, appointments, and decisions. Each step forward was marked by a new challenge—undergoing invasive tests, deciphering complex medical terms, and bracing for treatments known to wreak havoc on the body. But, with every decision, there was a resolve: to trust the medical professionals, to lean into the support of loved ones, and to endure every discomfort, every side effect, no matter how debilitating.

Facing the horizon of the upcoming medical journey, I felt an inner reservoir of strength bubbling up. While the path was undoubtedly paved with complexities—treatments, tests, and medical consultations—it also represented a beacon of hope, a bridge to recovery. With each step forward, I was not just confronting a diagnosis but actively championing my own well-being.

Attitude, I realized, would be the cornerstone of this journey. Choosing to face each day with optimism and courage would amplify the effectiveness of the treatments and shape my experience. Every dawn presented an opportunity to recommit to healing, to harness the innate strength that resides in all of us, and to face challenges head-on with resilience and hope.

With clarity on the road ahead and the unwavering support of loved ones and medical professionals, I felt prepared. Each treatment, each consultation, would not only be a measure against the disease but also a step towards reclaiming my health and vitality.

5

Who to Fight For?

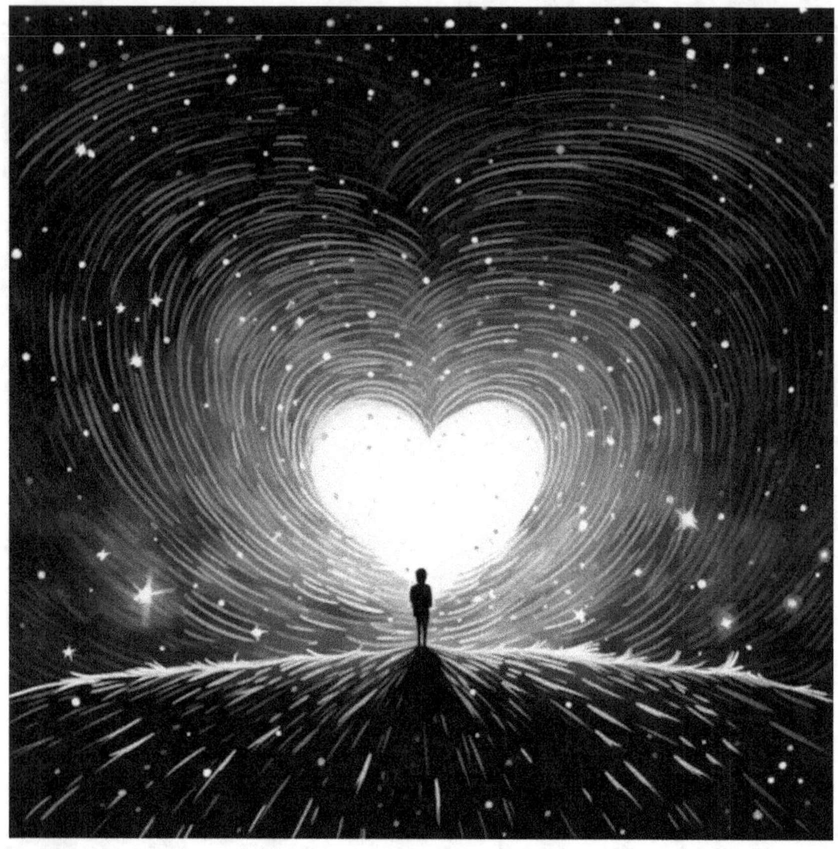

When faced with a challenge, a common question arises: Why am I doing this? Who am I doing it for? As I began my journey through cancer, these questions took center stage. It wasn't just about a medical diagnosis or a treatment plan; it was about understanding the reasons behind my will to overcome and move forward. This chapter delves into the driving forces in my life—the people who matter most to me and the realization of the importance of self-care and personal motivation. It's about recognizing the why behind the fight and understanding that sometimes, the most crucial reason to keep going is oneself.

Pillars in Life

Each of us, throughout our lives, builds foundations on which our spirits rest and draw strength. These foundations are often shaped by people, those rare souls whose love and presence anchor us, especially during tempestuous times. For me, those pillars were unmistakably my family. My children, with their contagious laughter and boundless curiosity, reminded me daily of the beauty of life and its endless possibilities. My wife, my unwavering partner in every chapter of our shared journey, provided strength in moments of weakness and hope in times of despair. My mother and sister, steadfast in their support, were the embodiment of familial love and sacrifice. And then there were the memories of those I'd lost—my father and grandmothers. Their legacy, the values they instilled, and the love they showered upon me became my guiding light, urging me to forge ahead with determination.

It's All for You

While these loved ones provided external strength and motivation, an internal reckoning emerged: the most significant reason to fight, to persevere, was for myself. This realization wasn't borne out of selfishness, but rather a profound understanding that self-love is the very essence of survival and well-being. Battling cancer wasn't just about reclaiming my life for the sake of others, but primarily for the life I owed to myself. If I was to be the protector, the provider, the beacon for my loved ones, I first needed to be whole, healthy, and present. This self-love wasn't merely about self-preservation but about honoring the commitment to the life I've been given. It reinforced that before I could pour love into the lives of others, I needed to ensure my own cup was full. This love for oneself, I realized, was the most potent weapon in my arsenal against cancer. It drove me to fight harder, heal faster, and emerge stronger, not just for my family, but fundamentally for the life I cherished and the future I envisioned.

At the heart of every battle, amidst the chaos and challenges, lies a profound truth. It's essential to understand that the love we hold for others is only as strong as the love we have for ourselves. By prioritizing our well-being, by valuing our existence, we not only enrich our lives but also enhance the lives of those around us. Each one of us has our cherished circle of family and friends, the faces that come to mind when we think of reasons to persevere. However, let's never forget that when we stand tall, when we embrace our worth, we illuminate the path not just for ourselves but for everyone who walks with us. The ultimate act of love, courage, and resilience is recognizing that the greatest reason to heal, to conquer any challenge, *IS YOU!*

6

The Faith

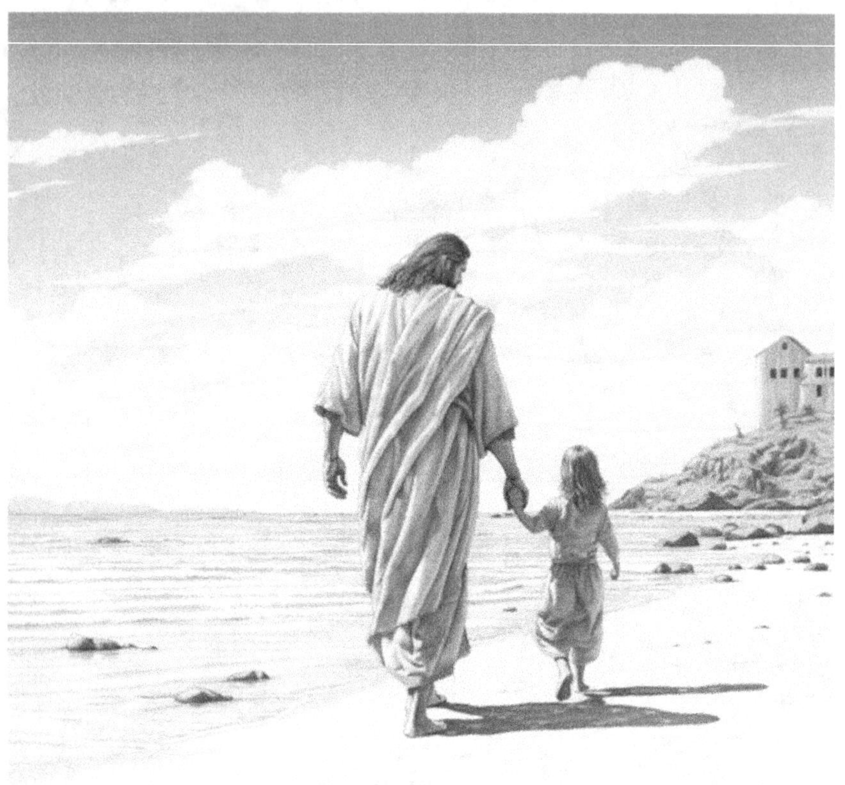

F aith can be understood as an unwavering trust, a belief in something greater than ourselves, often beyond tangible proof or understanding. It's this innate sense of hope and assurance, acting as an anchor during turbulent times. In the face of adversity, such as a daunting diagnosis like cancer, faith becomes an invaluable source of strength and resilience. Trusting in God's design, even amidst the mire of confusion and fear, can illuminate the path forward. It provides a framework for understanding, a belief that there's a larger purpose at play, even in the throes of suffering. Relying on God's wisdom and mercy, many find the courage to combat not just cancer, but any affliction, drawing strength from a divine wellspring that assures us we're never truly alone in our battles.

Religious Foundations of What You Believe

Faith is the anchor that grounds us when the storms of life threaten to sweep us away. For me, that unwavering faith has always been rooted in God's eternal love and promise. From a young age, I was taught to lean on Him, to turn to Him in prayer during moments of despair, and to seek His guidance when the path became uncertain.

One of the most profound stories that always resonated with me is about walking alongside God on a beach. In this narrative, as I journeyed through life, I noticed two sets of footprints in the sand, representing God walking beside me. However, during the toughest moments—times filled with doubt, pain, and fear—I observed just one set of footprints. Initially, this made me feel abandoned. How could God leave me when I felt most vulnerable? But, upon reflection, I came to a heartwarming realization. Those solitary footprints were not mine but God's. In those trying moments, He wasn't beside me; He was carrying me, cradling me in His arms, ensuring I wasn't facing my challenges alone.

The teachings, the scriptures, the prayers—all became the foundational pillars that held me firm. Especially in times of adversity, like confronting cancer, I found solace in God's word, in the belief that He has a grand plan, even if it is beyond my comprehension. I learned a valuable lesson: we must do what is humanly possible and trust that God will handle what's humanly impossible. This belief became my touchstone.

God's Timing is Perfect

It's natural to question, to wonder why certain things happen when they do, particularly when they shake the very core of our being. But in my journey with cancer, I came to realize that there's a divine timing in everything. While the human heart may rush or resist, God's clock runs on its own pace, ensuring that every event, every challenge, and every blessing unfolds precisely when it's meant to. It took introspection, patience, and immense faith to understand that my diagnosis, as tough as it was, came into my life at a specific moment for a reason. A reason that, with time, would bring clarity, growth, and deeper understanding.

The Biggest Fish is Not Caught on the Seashore

Every hardship we face in life is akin to a deep-sea expedition. While one can find small rewards close to the shore, the most significant treasures—the lessons that transform our soul and character—are found in the deeper, turbulent waters. Just as the angler knows that the largest, most rewarding catch demands venturing into the vast, open sea, I came to understand that life's most valuable lessons aren't found in the comfort of the shallow but in the challenges of the deep. This analogy rings true for life's challenges as well. The shallow waters of everyday life, with its minor irritations and fleeting joys, were familiar territory. But this diagnosis pushed me further out, away from the comfort of the known. It forced me to grapple with deeper questions, to confront fears I didn't know I had, and to discover strengths I never knew I possessed.

Confronting cancer was my voyage into these profound depths. It wasn't a journey I'd have chosen, but it was one that enriched me in ways I couldn't have imagined.

But here's the beauty of venturing into the deep: it's where the most significant growth occurs. Every challenge faced, every fear overcome, every pain relieved, added to my understanding of life and myself. It taught me about resilience, about the depth of human spirit, and about the incredible power of hope and faith. Just as the angler returns from the deep sea with tales of great battles and even greater catches, my journey through this ordeal enriched me with experiences and lessons that I wouldn't trade for anything. The deeper the waters, the more significant the lessons. And while the journey into the deep is filled with uncertainty and risks, it's also where the promise of true discovery and growth is. In God's grand design, He led me into deep waters. It was not to drown me, but a test of my faith, urging me to catch the most magnificent fish.

7

The Long Way to Go

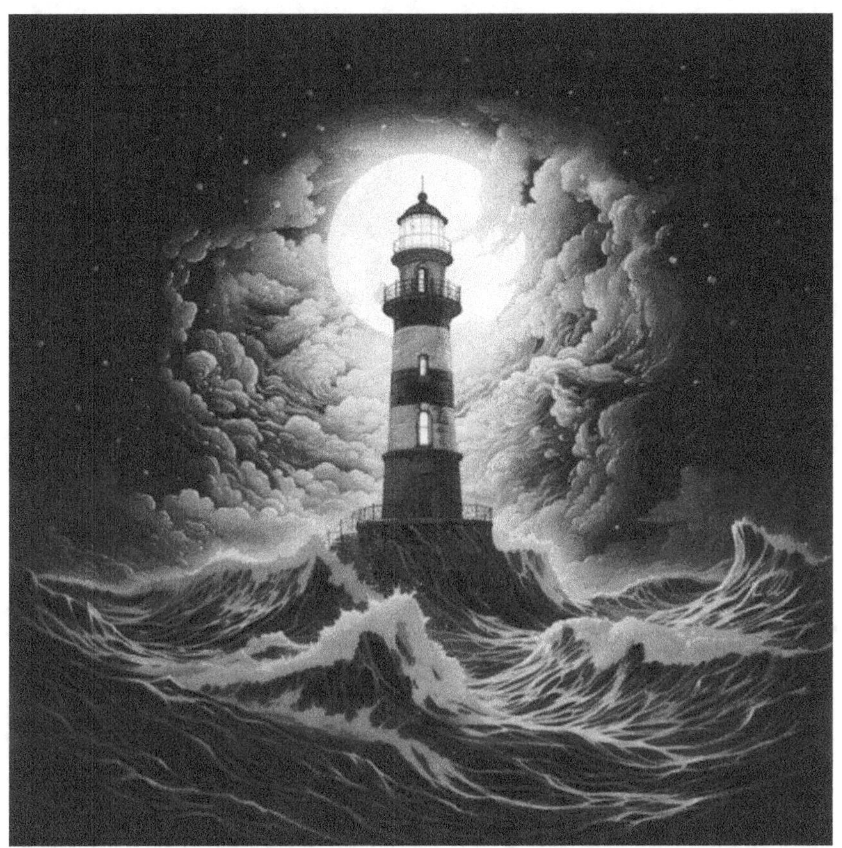

Confronting cancer is a marathon, demanding physical endurance, mental resilience, and emotional fortitude. A big portion of immediate concerns are physical. Treatments like chemotherapy and radiation, while effective, come with a range of side effects that can change daily routines. The body becomes both the battleground and the soldier, waging wars against mutating cells, enduring invasive procedures, and grappling with the side effects of aggressive treatments. Each day might bring a new symptom: fatigue that clings to the bones, pains that migrate without warning, or changes in appearance that mirror the internal struggle. But beyond the evident physical hardships, there are also significant mental and emotional challenges to address.

This chapter aims to shed light on the rigors and revelations of this journey, balancing the brutalities of medical treatments with the indomitable spirit of hope, the power of positivity and the anchoring strength of faith, and backed by personal insights and scientific evidence.

Medical Process Path

Cancer treatments are a rigorous endeavor, characterized by an array of symptoms that differ markedly between individuals. What one person experiences might not mirror another's journey, making it nearly impossible to draw direct comparisons. In fact, prior life challenges, no matter how demanding, seem almost small when placed against the weight of a cancer diagnosis.

The side effects of the treatments are varied and intense. Personally, I grappled with debilitating nausea, significant dryness affecting the skin and mucous membranes, heightened sensitivity in my mouth, metallic taste, and the evident changes in weight and hair loss. But as overwhelming as these symptoms were, the overarching objective remained clear: healing. The medicines, though aggressive in their nature, serve a dual purpose. They challenge the body but also pave the path to recovery. Amidst these challenges, there was a silver lining in my mindset. I began to perceive these symptoms as signals — a good sign that the medicines were indeed working, actively striving to heal my body.

Every symptom, as grueling as it was, became secondary to the ultimate goal of recovery. And this sentiment wasn't unique to me. In my journey, I encountered fellow fighters, some of whom bore even more significant scars, like the loss of a limb, but their spirit remained indomitable.

A notable memory from my treatment phase was during my initial chemotherapy session. Despite the discomfort, a sense of hope was shared by a woman seated beside me. She leaned over and candidly remarked, "*This process is painful, undeniably uncomfortable, and quite challenging; but hold on and be patient because It works!*". That sentiment became a beacon, reminding me that every symptom, every challenge was a step closer to healing.

Symptoms will fade, and you'll regain your weight and hair and even if some changes are lasting forever, you'll find new ways to enjoy life at every stage.

The imminent medical treatment phase, though daunting, was a pathway lined with expertise and care. A dedicated team of healthcare professionals, armed with knowledge and experience, stood ready to guide me through each phase. Their proficiency, combined with my determination, created a potent force against the ailment.

Modern Medical Treatments for Cancer: Triumphs of Science and Technology

In the dynamic landscape of medical science, our fight against cancer has been propelled by groundbreaking innovations and technological advances. Today, thanks to relentless research and development, patients have access to a range of treatments that not only enhance survival rates but also improve the quality of life. Here's a look at some of the latest, optimistic strides in cancer care:

1. **Targeted Therapy:** Moving beyond the traditional '*one-size-fits-all*' approach, targeted therapies are designed to target specific molecules and gene mutations that contribute to cancer growth. By focusing on these unique characteristics, these treatments aim to halt or slow the progression of cancer, ensuring minimal harm to

healthy cells.

2. **Robotic Surgery:** With the advent of robotics in medicine, surgeries have become more precise and minimally invasive. This technology allows surgeons to operate with enhanced vision, precision, and control, ensuring faster recovery and reduced hospitalization.

3. **Immunotherapy:** This revolutionary treatment harnesses the power of the body's own immune system to fight cancer. By boosting the immune response or introducing lab-engineered immune system proteins, immunotherapy can effectively target and destroy cancer cells.

4. **Precision Medicine:** Tailored to the genetic makeup of each patient, precision medicine offers treatments based on the genetic changes in one's cancer cells. This ensures that patients receive treatments that are most likely to provide benefits, minimizing side effects.

5. **Proton Therapy:** An advanced form of radiation therapy, proton therapy uses protons instead of X-rays to treat cancer. This ensures that radiation is delivered with extreme precision, targeting the tumor while sparing surrounding healthy tissues.

6. **Nano-medicine:** At the intersection of nanotechnology and medicine, nano-medicine offers the promise of delivering drugs directly to cancer cells. This not only enhances the effectiveness of treatment but also significantly reduces potential side effects.

7. **3D Conformal Radiation Therapy:** Using advanced technology to map the shape of the tumor, this therapy ensures that radiation beams are shaped precisely to the tumor, protecting nearby organs and tissues.

These treatments, and many more in the pipeline, underscore the relentless spirit of science and technology in the quest to conquer cancer. With each passing day, we move closer to transforming cancer from a formidable foe into a manageable condition, all thanks to the wonders of modern medicine. The future for cancer care is brighter than ever, offering hope and healing to countless individuals worldwide.

Where the Mind Leads, the Body Achieves

The centrality of the mind in the journey of healing cannot be under-stated. Time and again, medical research has underscored the profound connection between a positive mindset and the body's capacity to heal. This isn't just about feeling good emotionally; it's about how our mental state can directly influence our physiological responses and, consequently, our recovery trajectory.

A positive mind releases a cascade of beneficial hormones, like endor-phins, which not only reduce the perception of pain but also enhance the body's immune responses. Conversely, persistent negative thoughts and stress can release cortisol, a hormone that, in prolonged excess, can suppress the immune system, making recovery more challenging.

In the realm of oncology, the mind's role is even more pronounced. Patients with a hopeful and positive outlook have been observed to experience better treatment outcomes. This isn't merely coincidental. A resilient mind can lead to better sleep, improved appetite, and overall better adherence to medical recommendations—all crucial elements in the cancer recovery process.

Thus, as we confront the challenges that come with a cancer diagnosis, equipping ourselves with a fortified mental stance becomes as crucial as any medical regimen. The mind, with its vast power, doesn't just complement the healing process; it actively drives it, making the journey towards recovery not just possible, but more probable.

The act of visualizing positive outcomes, of fostering hope, and of surrounding oneself with optimism isn't just about mental well-being. It serves as an essential catalyst that propels the body towards healing.

Every thought, every burst of positivity, and every moment of hope sends signals to our cells, promoting repair and rejuvenation.

Stress and Negative Thoughts versus Positive Thought and Long-Term Vision

In the face of daunting challenges like cancer, the mental environment we cultivate becomes paramount. Negative thoughts, pessimistic comments, and distressing news can act as detrimental forces, potentially hindering the healing process. There's a mounting body of evidence suggesting that prolonged exposure to stress and negativity can exacerbate physical ailments and dampen the immune response. However, seeking positive emotions isn't about suppressing the negative ones. It's crucial to acknowledge and process all emotions, but it's equally vital to create moments that invite positivity. This might mean reconnecting with a hobby, watching a heartwarming movie, spending quality time with loved ones, or simply taking a moment to appreciate the beauty of a sunrise.

On the other hand, fostering a positive mindset and envisioning a brighter, long-term future can act as catalysts for recovery. By maintaining a forward-looking vision, whether it's seeing children graduate, celebrating milestones with loved ones, or achieving personal goals, the mind establishes a beacon of hope and purpose. This perspective doesn't just offer emotional solace; it actively contributes to physical well-being.

It's essential, then, to be conscious of the environment and the influences we allow into our lives. Surrounding oneself with optimistic individuals, uplifting stories, and affirmative experiences can be a transformative strategy. In essence, while medical treatments tackle the physical aspects of the disease, a positive environment and a hopeful vision work in tandem to heal the spirit, offering a comprehensive approach to overcoming cancer.

In my personal journey, mental tenacity was anchored in the future I envisioned. The thought of watching my two children grow and thrive, of sharing countless moments and memories with my wife and family, fortified my resolve. Additionally, visualizing my future projects and ambitions gave me a direction and purpose, reinforcing the belief that overcoming cancer was not just possible, but probable. These visions of the future not only offered solace during challenging times but also kindled a fire to continue the fight, instilling a deep-seated belief that I had many more years ahead.

Everyone's source of strength is unique. Actively setting the mind on and visualizing one's projects and aspirations for the future has been shown to be a potent tool in the battle against cancer. Whether it's looking forward to events 40 years down the line, or merely anticipating the joys of the next 2 years or 2 months, these anchors play a pivotal role. Keeping them at the forefront can act as a shield, warding off negative thoughts and fortifying one's mental resilience. In the battle against cancer, having such mental anchors, combined with scientific advances, creates a formidable strategy to overcome the toughest challenges.

8

Rebuilding the Body

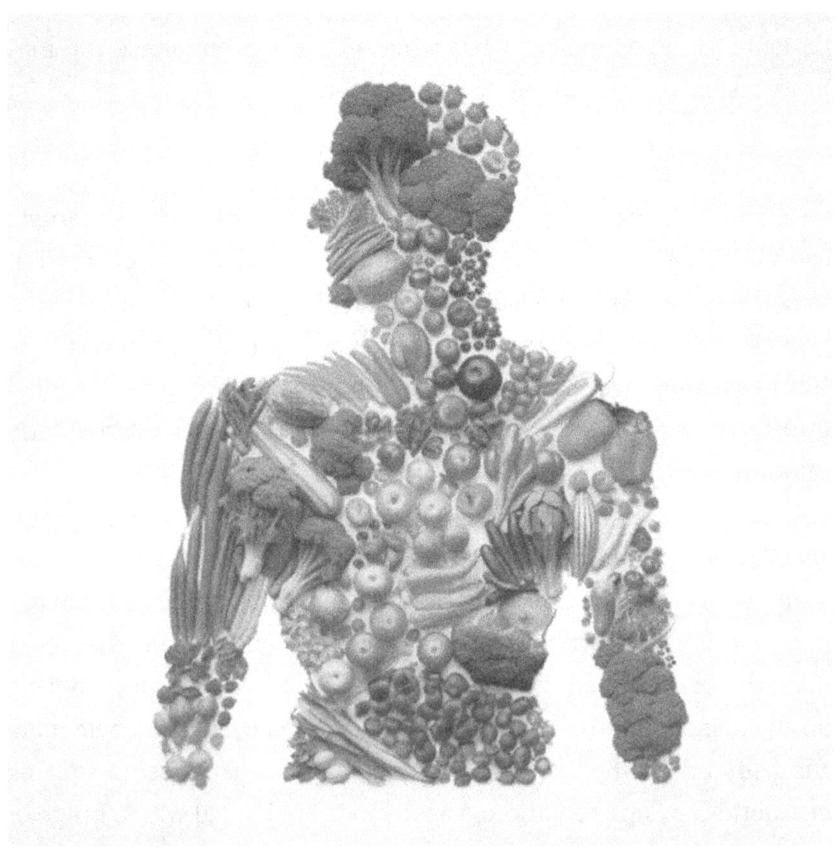

For those battling cancer, it isn't just about the medical treatments. Equally important, if not more, is the role of nutrition, physical activity, and a proper sleep routine in healing and recovery. Let's delve into the scientific realm to understand why and how these elements are crucial, offering practical and actionable advice along the way.

Eat to beat! Optimizing nutrition, understanding the basics.

Nutrition and Cancer

Diet plays a pivotal role in the overall health and recovery of cancer patients. Studies indicate that what we eat can influence the risk, progression, and overall outcome of cancer.

Optimal Nutrition During Chemotherapy

Chemotherapy is a rigorous medical treatment, and while it targets cancer cells, it can also impact healthy cells and lead to side effects that may interfere with one's ability to eat and absorb nutrients. Proper nutrition can help patients maintain their strength, prevent body tissue from breaking down, rebuild tissue, and maintain defenses against infection. Among the nutrients, protein stands out as particularly important.

The Power of Plant-Based Foods in the Fight Against Cancer

For individuals diagnosed with cancer, a robust nutrition plan becomes paramount in supporting treatment, recovery, and overall well-being. Plant-based foods emerge as potent allies during this journey, offering an abundance of nutrients and compounds that can aid in strengthening the body and combating the adverse effects of treatments such as chemotherapy and radiation. These foods are loaded with a range of antioxidants, phytochemicals, and fibers that work in multiple ways to protect our cells and encourage their healthy growth.

1. **Rich in Phytochemicals:** Plant-based foods are abundant in phytochemicals—natural compounds that have been shown to slow the growth of cancer cells and reduce inflammation. Examples include flavonoids in berries, curcumin in turmeric, and sulforaphane in cruciferous vegetables.

2. **Natural Antioxidants:** Antioxidants found in fruits, vegetables, nuts, and seeds help neutralize harmful free radicals in the body, supporting cellular health. For instance, vitamin C from citrus fruits, vitamin E from nuts and seeds, and beta-carotene from car-

rots and sweet potatoes can all contribute to antioxidant defenses.

3. **Essential Fibers:** Plant-based foods, particularly whole grains and legumes, are excellent sources of dietary fiber. Fiber aids in digestion, reduces constipation—a common side effect of some cancer treatments—and supports a healthy gut microbiome, which plays a role in immune function.

4. **Source of Vital Nutrients:** Many cancer patients might experience deficiencies in specific vitamins and minerals. Plant-based foods, such as leafy greens, nuts, seeds, and whole grains, are packed with essential nutrients like iron, magnesium, potassium, and B-vitamins, which support energy production and overall cellular functions.

5. **Low in Saturated Fat:** Plant-based diets are typically lower in saturated fats. While fats are essential for energy, especially during cancer treatment, focusing on healthy fats from plants like avocados, nuts, and olives can be beneficial.

6. **Alkaline-promoting Foods:** Some believe that an alkaline diet can help reduce the acidity in the body and thus hinder cancer cell growth. While scientific evidence is ongoing, many plant-based foods, including green leafy vegetables, are considered alkaline-promoting.

7. **Hydration:** Fruits like watermelon, cucumber, and oranges have high water content. Proper hydration is crucial during cancer treatment to help flush out toxins, combat fatigue, and maintain healthy skin.

Examples of Power-Packed Plant Foods for Cancer Patients:

Vegetables

- **Cruciferous Vegetables:** Broccoli, cauliflower, Brussels sprouts, and kale are rich in sulforaphane, which has demonstrated potential anti-cancer properties. They contain glucosinolates, which in the body convert to compounds that help in the elimination of carcinogens.
- **Leafy Greens:** Spinach, kale, and collard greens are packed with fiber, folate, and a range of antioxidants.
- **Garlic:** Part of the allium family of vegetables, garlic has been found to have cancer-treatment properties, especially related to the digestive system.

Fruits

- **Berries:** Blueberries, strawberries, and raspberries contain antioxidants and phytochemicals that can support cellular health.
- **Citrus Fruits:** Oranges, grapefruits, and lemons contain flavonoids which may inhibit the growth of cancer cells and stop the spread of tumors.
- **Tomatoes:** They have lycopene, a powerful antioxidant that has been linked to a reduced risk of prostate cancer.

Whole Grains: Foods like quinoa, oats, and brown rice provide essential nutrients and dietary fiber.

- **Quinoa:** A complete protein and packed with antioxidants.
- **Brown Rice:** Contains natural fiber which helps in detoxifying the body. Fiber assists the body in eliminating waste, which can sometimes contain harmful agents.
- **Oats:** Contain a type of fiber called beta-glucan which can lower the risk of colorectal cancer.

Legumes: Lentils, chickpeas, and beans are excellent protein sources, offering an alternative to animal proteins.

Seeds and Nuts: Flaxseeds, chia seeds, walnuts, and almonds provide essential fatty acids, protein, and antioxidants.

- **Flaxseeds:** Rich in omega-3 fatty acids and lignans, which have antioxidant properties.
- **Walnuts:** Contain polyphenols that can suppress the growth of breast and prostate cancer cells.

Incorporating a wide variety of plant-based foods can help nourish the body, alleviate some treatment side effects, and support recovery. By consuming a broad array of fruits, vegetables, whole grains, nuts, and seeds, you can ensure you're getting a comprehensive mix of the antioxidants, phytochemicals, and fibers that contribute to their protective effects.

One of the most important things to remember when incorporating plant-based foods into a cancer-fighting diet is variety. Different plant foods offer different types and amounts of key nutrients and beneficial compounds. While a plant-based diet offers numerous benefits, it's essential to work with a healthcare professional or nutritionist who can provide tailored advice based on individual needs and treatment plans.

The Importance of Protein During Chemotherapy

Protein is vital for many functions in the body. It is essential for growth, tissue repair, immune function, and the maintenance of lean body mass. During chemotherapy:

1. **Tissue Repair:** Chemotherapy can cause damage to healthy cells. Protein helps in the repair of tissues in the body, aiding recovery.
2. **Immune Function:** A sufficient intake of protein is crucial for the

synthesis of immune cells and antibodies, which help the body fight off infections—a common concern during chemotherapy.

3. **Maintaining Muscle Mass:** Chemotherapy can lead to muscle wasting due to reduced appetite or other side effects. Adequate protein intake can help prevent excessive muscle loss.

Foods to Boost Protein Intake During Chemotherapy

- **Lean Meats:** Chicken, turkey, and lean cuts of beef or pork are rich sources of protein.
- **Fish:** Oily fish like salmon, mackerel, and sardines not only provide protein but also beneficial omega-3 fatty acids.
- **Eggs:** They are versatile, easily digestible, and packed with protein.
- **Dairy Products:** Greek yogurt, cottage cheese, and milk are good choices. For those who are lactose intolerant, lactose-free options are available.
- **Legumes:** Lentils, chickpeas, and beans are not only protein-rich but also provide a good amount of fiber.
- **Tofu and Tempeh:** These soy-based products are excellent protein sources and can be incorporated into various dishes.
- **Seeds and Nuts:** Almonds, walnuts, chia seeds, and flaxseeds can be sprinkled on salads, yogurt, or consumed as snacks for a protein boost.
- **Whole Grains:** Foods like quinoa and oats can be a significant protein source, especially for those following a vegetarian or vegan diet.

The Imperative of Adequate Water Consumption during Cancer Treatment

Water plays an indispensable role in the overall health and well-being of cancer patients. As the primary component of our cells, tissues, and organs, water is fundamental for almost every metabolic process in the body. During cancer treatment, the body undergoes increased metabolic activity, and the need for proper hydration intensifies. Adequate water intake aids in flushing out toxins and waste products, which are often elevated due to treatments like chemotherapy. Moreover, several cancer medications and therapies can lead to dehydration, making it essential for patients to consume additional fluids. Proper hydration also alleviates symptoms like dry mouth and constipation, common side effects of cancer treatments. Furthermore, maintaining optimal water balance can combat fatigue, improve cognitive function, and support the body's natural healing processes. Given the rigorous physical and emotional challenges that cancer patients face, ensuring consistent and adequate water intake becomes a vital aspect of their holistic care.

Other Nutritional Considerations During Chemotherapy

While protein is fundamental, other aspects of nutrition are equally important during chemotherapy:

1. **Caloric Intake:** During cancer treatment, the body often faces heightened energy demands as it works diligently to repair cells, combat the disease, and withstand the taxing effects of treatments like chemotherapy and radiation. This increased need for energy makes it essential to ensure sufficient calorie intake. Consuming nutrient-dense foods such as avocados, nuts, whole grains, lean proteins like chicken or fish, and natural fats like olive oil can help meet these caloric requirements. By integrating these healthy options, patients can not only maintain body weight and muscle mass but also gain the strength and endurance needed to endure treatment and bolster recovery afterward.

2. **Minimizing Processed Foods:** Avoiding overly processed foods, high in sugars, or charred, is crucial in cancer treatment because these foods often contain harmful additives, preservatives, and

artificial ingredients that can exacerbate inflammation and hinder the body's natural healing processes, in addition to their potential carcinogenic properties. Processed foods are also typically low in essential nutrients and high in sugars, unhealthy fats, and empty calories. These components can compromise the immune system, making it less effective in combating cancer cells. Embracing a diet rich in whole, unprocessed foods ensures that the body receives the vital nutrients it needs to support recovery and overall well-being during cancer treatment.

3. **Avoiding tobacco and alcohol:** Following a cancer diagnosis, it's crucial to make informed choices to support the healing journey. Patients should ideally avoid tobacco and alcohol consumption, both of which can exacerbate health concerns and potentially interfere with treatments.

4. **Overexposure to the sun:** During cancer treatment, particularly chemotherapy and radiation, the skin can become more sensitive and vulnerable. This heightened sensitivity means that the skin is more susceptible to the damaging effects of the sun's ultraviolet (UV) rays. Prolonged exposure can result in severe sunburns, even with minimal sun exposure. Additionally, certain chemotherapy drugs can make the skin more photosensitive, leading to quicker and more intense sunburn reactions. It's crucial for individuals undergoing cancer treatment to take extra precautions, such as wearing sunscreen, protective clothing, and avoiding peak sun hours, to reduce the risk of skin damage and potential complications.

Tailored Nutritional Approaches:

Different cancer types, stages, and treatment methods can require specific dietary considerations. Here are tailored nutritional approaches based on specific cancer scenarios:

Breast Cancer:

- **Phytoestrogens:** Found in foods like flaxseeds and soy products, they can have an estrogen-like effect on the body, which might be beneficial or harmful depending on the type of breast cancer.
- **Cruciferous Vegetables:** Broccoli, Brussels sprouts, and cauliflower contain compounds that might help to fight cancer cells.

Colorectal Cancer:

- **High Fiber:** Whole grains, fruits, and vegetables can help in promoting healthy bowel movements and might decrease the risk of recurrence.
- **Limit Red Meat:** Excessive consumption might be associated with an increased risk of colorectal cancer.

Prostate Cancer:

- **Tomatoes:** Rich in lycopene, which has been linked to reduced risk of prostate cancer.
- **Green Tea:** Contains polyphenols which might help in slowing down the progression of prostate cancer.

Lung Cancer:

- **Cruciferous Vegetables:** These can be particularly beneficial.
- **Vitamin-rich Fruits:** Oranges, berries, and kiwi can provide essential vitamins and antioxidants.

Stomach/Gastric Cancer:

- **Limit Salted & Pickled Foods:** High consumption can be a risk factor.
- **Consume Fresh Fruits & Vegetables:** They can provide essential nutrients and help in preventing irritation in the stomach.

Pancreatic Cancer:

- **Limit Alcohol and Fatty Foods:** They can exacerbate symptoms or risks.
- **Consume Easy-to-digest Meals:** Opt for smaller, frequent meals that are low in fat but rich in nutrients.

It's also essential to steer clear of unverified alternative therapies or supplements without consulting the oncologist, as these might negatively interact with prescribed treatments or offer false hopes.

In summary, while undergoing chemotherapy, it's paramount to maintain a balanced diet. However, it's essential to remember that individual needs can vary based on the type of chemotherapy, its side effects, and other individual factors. Working with a registered dietitian who specializes in oncology nutrition can provide personalized guidance and recommendations.

Let's get physical.

The Science Behind Movement: Regular physical activity is known to boost the immune system, improve mood by releasing endorphins, and reduce the risk of chronic diseases. Studies showed that regular physical activity could reduce the risk of breast and colon cancers.

Post-Diagnosis Activity: Paving the Road to Recovery
Once a cancer diagnosis is made, integrating physical activity into

daily life becomes even more crucial. Exercise can serve as a means to boost energy, alleviate some of the side effects of treatment, and most importantly, improve overall quality of life. While the thought of exercising might feel daunting initially, understanding the profound benefits and taking gradual steps can make the journey easier.

1. **Boosting Energy:** Paradoxically, physical activity can help combat the fatigue often associated with cancer treatments. A moderate exercise routine, even simple activities like walking or light stretching, can significantly boost energy levels, counteracting the fatigue induced by treatments like chemotherapy or radiation.

2. **Enhancing Mood:** Physical activity stimulates the release of endorphins, the body's natural mood elevators. This can be a valuable tool in combating the emotional roller coaster that often accompanies a cancer diagnosis, providing mental clarity and uplifting the spirit.

3. **Improving Treatment Efficiency:** Some studies have shown that physically active cancer patients might respond better to treatments. Regular exercise can improve cardiovascular health and lung capacity, potentially enhancing the body's ability to process and recover from various treatments.

4. **Maintaining Muscle Mass & Bone Density:** Cancer treatments can lead to muscle wasting and reduced bone density. Engaging in resistance training, even with light weights or resistance bands, can help maintain muscle mass and protect bone health.

5. **Improving Balance and Reducing Fall Risk:** Especially important for individuals undergoing treatments that can affect balance or for those on medications that might cause dizziness. Simple balance exercises, like standing on one foot or walking heel-to-toe, can be beneficial.

6. **Optimizing Immune Function:** Moderate exercise can give a

notable boost to the immune system, potentially enhancing the body's ability to ward off infections during a time when it's most vulnerable.

Practical Ways to Start:

- **Walking:** Starting with short distances and gradually increasing as energy and stamina allow.
- **Yoga:** Gentle poses can improve flexibility, strength, and mindfulness.
- **Pilates:** Focuses on core strength, which is crucial for overall stability.
- **Resistance Training:** Using light weights or resistance bands to maintain muscle mass.
- **Swimming:** A low-impact exercise that offers resistance for muscle strength while being gentle on the joints.

A Word of Caution: It's essential to consult with healthcare professionals before beginning or modifying any exercise regimen post-diagnosis. They can provide guidelines tailored to individual circumstances, ensuring safety and maximizing benefits. Listening to one's body, understanding limits, and making modifications as needed is crucial.

Sleep Well: The Foundation for Healing

Sleep plays a pivotal role in the healing and recovery process, especially for cancer patients. It's during these hours of rest that the body repairs itself, strengthening the immune system, detoxifying, and rejuvenating both physically and mentally.

Benefits of Quality Sleep:

- **Cellular Repair and Growth:** During deep sleep, the body releases growth hormones that facilitate cell regeneration, crucial for repairing the damage caused by cancer treatments.
- **Enhanced Immune Function:** Consistent, restful sleep strengthens the immune system, aiding the body in warding off infections and supporting its fight against cancer.
- **Mental Health and Cognitive Function:** Adequate sleep improves mood, reduces anxiety and depression, and enhances cognitive functions, helping patients cope better with their diagnosis and treatment.
- **Metabolic Regulation:** Sleep helps regulate the hormones that control appetite, which can be crucial for maintaining a healthy weight during and after treatment.
- **Detoxification:** During sleep, the brain actively clears out toxins, a process especially important when the body is processing medications and treatments.

Tips for Improving Sleep Quality:

1. **Consistent Sleep Schedule:** Going to bed and waking up at the same time daily helps regulate the body's internal clock, promoting better sleep.
2. **Cool, Dark, and Quiet Environment:** These conditions are conducive to sleep. Consider using blackout curtains, earplugs, or a white noise machine if necessary.
3. **Limit Screen Time:** The blue light emitted by phones, tablets, and computers can interfere with melatonin production, a hormone responsible for sleep. It's advisable to limit screen exposure at least an hour before bed.
4. **Limit Caffeine and Alcohol:** Both can disrupt the sleep cycle, so consider reducing intake, especially in the hours leading up to

bedtime.

5. **Relaxation Techniques:** Activities like reading, deep breathing exercises, or meditation can help calm the mind, preparing it for sleep.

6. **Comfortable Bedding:** Ensure that mattresses and pillows are comfortable and supportive.

7. **Seek Professional Help:** Consulting a sleep specialist or therapist. They can provide strategies or treatments tailored to individual needs.

For cancer patients, restful sleep isn't just a matter of comfort; it's a cornerstone of the recovery process. Prioritizing sleep and adopting habits to promote better rest can significantly enhance the healing journey, supporting both the body and mind during this challenging time.

In the battle against cancer, it's a multidimensional approach that ensures the best outcome. While medical treatments address the disease, proper nutrition, physical activity, and good sleep help in rebuilding and rejuvenating the body. Harness the power of these natural healers, backed by science, to pave the path to recovery.

9

A Stroke of Gratitude

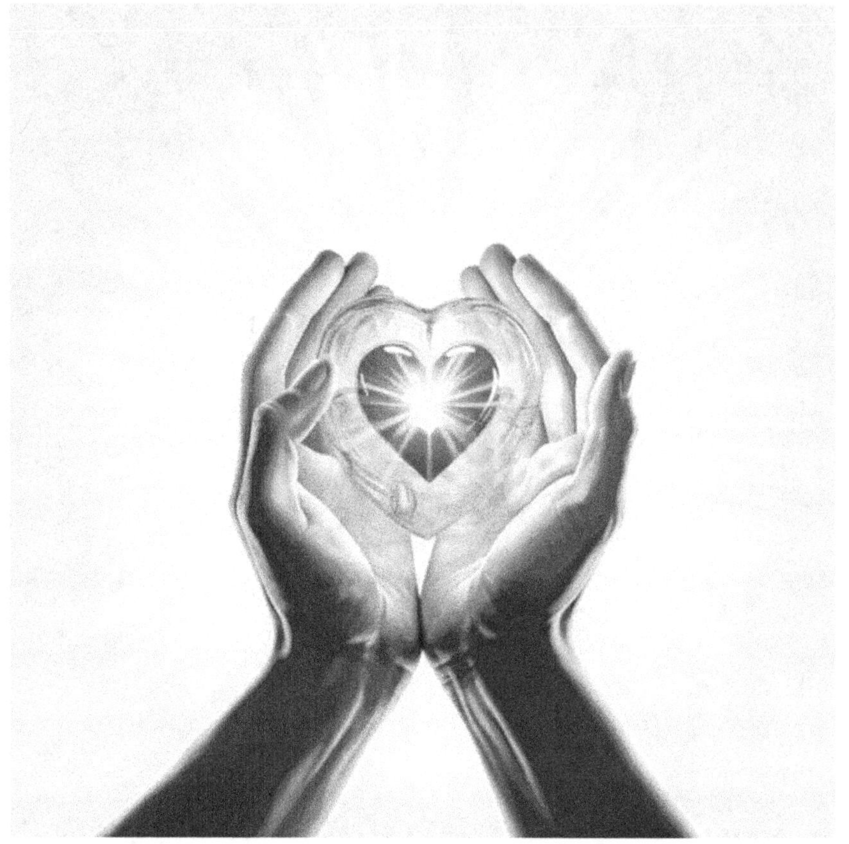

When we are faced with the absolute unimaginable, our perceptions are warped, mired in shadows. In those dark moments, as I found myself tumbling down the abyss of a cancer diagnosis, it was faith that caught me—a net woven by hands both divine and mortal.

In the hushed stillness of every night and the dawning light of every day, my heart wells up with an ineffable gratitude to the Divine. It was God's guiding hand that steered me through the tempestuous seas of my diagnosis and treatment. In moments of unbearable fear, pain and uncertainty, it was His whispers of hope and love that I clung to. Every glimmer of hope, every instance of healing, I see as a testament to His boundless mercy and grace. It wasn't just about the physical healing; it was the spiritual fortitude, the daily renewal of faith, and the inexplicable peace amidst the storm that became my anchors. This journey with cancer was not just a battle against a disease but a profound journey closer to Him. And for that, my heart overflows with gratitude.

Where does the love come from?

In the raw vulnerability that cancer exposed me to, I discovered the profound depths of love. Every prayer whispered in my name, every comforting hand on my shoulder, and every act of faith was testament to that. My gratitude for God's presence during this turbulent phase of my life is boundless, as it was from Him that the streams of love flowed—from family, friends, and well-wishers.

My wife, the beacon during my darkest nights, stood unwavering. The tenderness she displayed, attending to my needs, soothing my fears— convinced me that everything was going to be fine and that all aggressive medicines entering to my body were furiously acting to heal me. She wore many hats - my nurse, my confidante, my biggest cheerleader, my eternal love. But above all, she was a constant reminder of love's healing power. In her eyes, I found reasons to fight, to get up every day, and to believe in a brighter tomorrow. She transformed our home into a haven, ensuring every detail catered to my comfort and healing. Her strength during this period was awe-inspiring, how she managed to hold together our world while her own heart was breaking is a testament to her unparalleled resilience and faith.

My mother, embodying strength and courage, portrayed resilience like I'd never seen before. How painful it must be for a mother to watch her son suffer and yet, she held strong for me. She, with her own triumphant journey against cancer, illuminated the path for me to conquer the same battle; She also taught me that some things are beyond our control and must be accepted with resignation and unwavering faith in God and regardless of how much time you've lived, there will be always something new challenging us, new battles to win; my lovely mother, living proof of an endless strength and source of love for children.

My sister, the vigilant guardian, ensured that the medical guardianship I received was nothing short of the best; I owe her more than I could ever imagine, thanks to my sister's cares, cancer was diagnosed to me at an early stage. She has carried the great weight of ensuring the health of the entire family; my gratitude for being my primary and loved Doctor and for her endless devotion to family love. Her constant motivation and love helped me strengthen my faith.

The imprints of those who've passed on, like my father, my very first real-life hero, and my loving grandmothers, remain deeply etched in my heart. Their memories serve as constant reminders of where I come from and the legacy I hope to pass on. Every decision, every step, carries a piece of their wisdom and love. In moments of stillness, I often feel their guiding presence, nudging me towards becoming the best version of myself. Their lives, though no longer physically present, continue to influence and inspire my path forward.

And my 2 children? Their love, pure and untainted, became my greatest inspiration to get out of bed, stand up and keep fighting. Their innocence and infinite love became my most powerful medicines, bringing hope and light into the darkest recesses of my journey. Every giggle, every touch, every simple "*I love you*", infused me with a vigor to fight, to heal, to return to them as the pillar they've always known. They were my reminders of life's beauty amidst the pain, the symbols of a future filled with memories yet to be made. Their presence was my rallying cry, pushing me forward, reminding me daily of the profound reasons I had to heal.

It's not about '*getting rid of*' the difficult stories but instead truly seeing them, owning them, and using them. This cancer journey has been my '*hard story*', and it helped me discern what truly mattered. The news today paints life as expendable, a painful irony when set against the furious struggles many of us face, simply wishing for a few more moments of existence. But, life, with all its imperfections, is breathtakingly beautiful. It's vital to declutter our lives of negativity, holding on to only those things that add value, spark joy, and bring meaning.

The chemotherapies, symptoms, and fear—they do leave scars, but these scars can be beautiful, becoming emblems of our tenacity, endurance, and the transformative power of positivity. They can be reminders of our strength and resilience. Only by embracing joy, love, and gratitude can we truly heal, both mentally and physically.

Joy, hope, love, gratitude, and amusement serve as catalysts that can transform despair into determination. They remind us of the beauty that still exists, even when our immediate surroundings appear bleak. By leaning into these emotions, we're not only improving our psychological well-being but also fostering an environment that supports physical healing.

Everyone has somebody to help!

There's a solidarity in suffering, an unspoken bond forged in shared adversity. When you've peered into the same abyss, you understand the depth of another's pain. Every individual diagnosed with cancer becomes part of a fraternity—a silent understanding, an unspoken camaraderie. It's an experience that binds us, making us yearn to stretch out a hand in help, in understanding, in love.

Sharing my experience of overcoming cancer with those currently in the throes of their battle is not just an act of kindness, but also one of fairness. One of the most profound ways to express my gratitude for the immense support I received during my cancer journey is to extend that same compassion and aid to others navigating their paths to recovery.

Just as I leaned on the stories, advice, and support of others during my most challenging moments, it's only right that I pay forward that lifeline.

By sharing my experiences, knowledge, and understanding, I can offer solace, guidance, and strength to those grappling with the uncertainty and challenges of their own battles. In doing so, I not only honor those who stood by me but also create a ripple effect of kindness and hope for someone else. It's a cycle of mutual support. Gratitude isn't just a feeling but an action, and by assisting others in their fight against cancer, I am truly embodying the spirit of thankfulness.

10

The Reason Why!

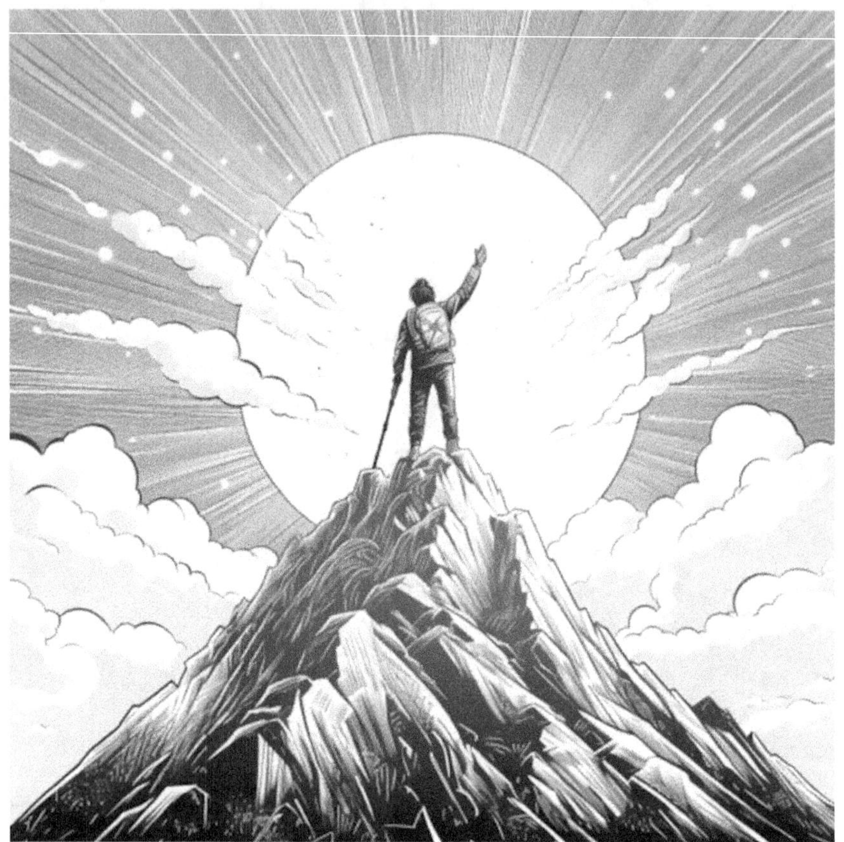

In life, every stroke of difficulty and challenge has an inherent purpose. We often move through life believing we're the architects of our destiny, crafting our futures with deliberate intent. But what happens when the universe, or more accurately, God's design, interrupts and redraws our plans?

When we're confronted with profound challenges, it's natural to question the purpose behind it all. Why me? Why this? Why now? Yet, as I learned after undergoing 14 chemotherapies and 2 surgeries to defeat colon and prostate cancer, there's a higher power at play, ensuring we find our way. I stand today as a testament to God's miracles and His infinite compassion and boundless mercy. It's a proof that even in the face of immense adversity, He doesn't burden us more than we can handle. Nature is a testament to His profound precision; not even a leaf sways without His consent.

Life isn't merely about existence, heartbeat and breath. It's about pursuing happiness, even amidst our flaws and imperfections. Often, we chase after happiness where is not, in the tangible – in wealth, accolades, and fleeting pleasures. However, the true essence of joy often resides in the intangible moments: a genuine smile exchanged, the warmth of a hug, the golden hues of a sunset, or the cathartic release of tears. It's found in the soft whisper of "*I love you*," the humility in "*I'm sorry*," the grace in "*I forgive you*," and the sincerity of "*thank you*." True happiness is molding ourselves into the people we aspire to be, irrespective of the time we believe we have left on this Earth.

From near death to truly healing

In the quiet corridors of hospitals and the long nights following chemotherapy and surgeries, I discovered the depths of my strength and resilience. I transitioned from moments of despair to moments of profound gratitude and faith. This journey wasn't just about combating a disease, a fight against an ailment of a cellular disorder; it was -and still is- about finding myself and experiencing God's limitless love and miracles.

With every chemotherapy session, every doctor's visit, and every prayer, there was an underlying hope—a hope that was more potent than the malignancy within. This journey taught me that healing doesn't just involve physical recovery. It's also a deep, emotional and spiritual revival where one learns to trust again, to hope more fiercely, and to cherish every breath. My story is a testament that our bodies and souls are capable of healing, and in that process, we can discover a renewed purpose and zest for life. Every scar, every tear, is a reminder that we can move from the brink of despair to profound gratitude, from near death to truly living.

Yet, here I am, not just a survivor but a testament to hope and resilience. I overcame cancer, and this victory isn't solely mine. It stands as a beacon for everyone who's battling this illness, proclaiming that every battle fought is a step closer to victory. *You can beat cancer too!*

Embrace the strength within you; believe that you too can conquer cancer and shine brighter than ever before!

Reborn to be me

The diagnosis was like an intense storm, testing the foundation of my existence. But in that tempest, something beautiful emerged—a rebirth of my spirit. Battling cancer didn't merely challenge my body; it ignited a profound transformation within.

I was compelled to re-evaluate my goals, my desires, and my dreams. Every moment of fear and pain also became an opportunity to discern what truly mattered. Stripped of pretenses and societal expectations, I found an authentic version of myself that had been waiting for recognition. This wasn't just about surviving a disease; it was about discovering an enriched identity—one forged in adversity but defined by hope, faith, and an unwavering zest for life.

We must not just live. We must live with intention, passion, and gratitude. I embrace each day as a gift, cherishing moments, both big and small, with renewed wonder. Every challenge has sculpted me, every tear has purified me, and every prayer has strengthened me. Today, I stand as a testament to the belief that we can rebuild, reform, and reimagine ourselves, always under the watchful and loving gaze of God.

11

Conclusion

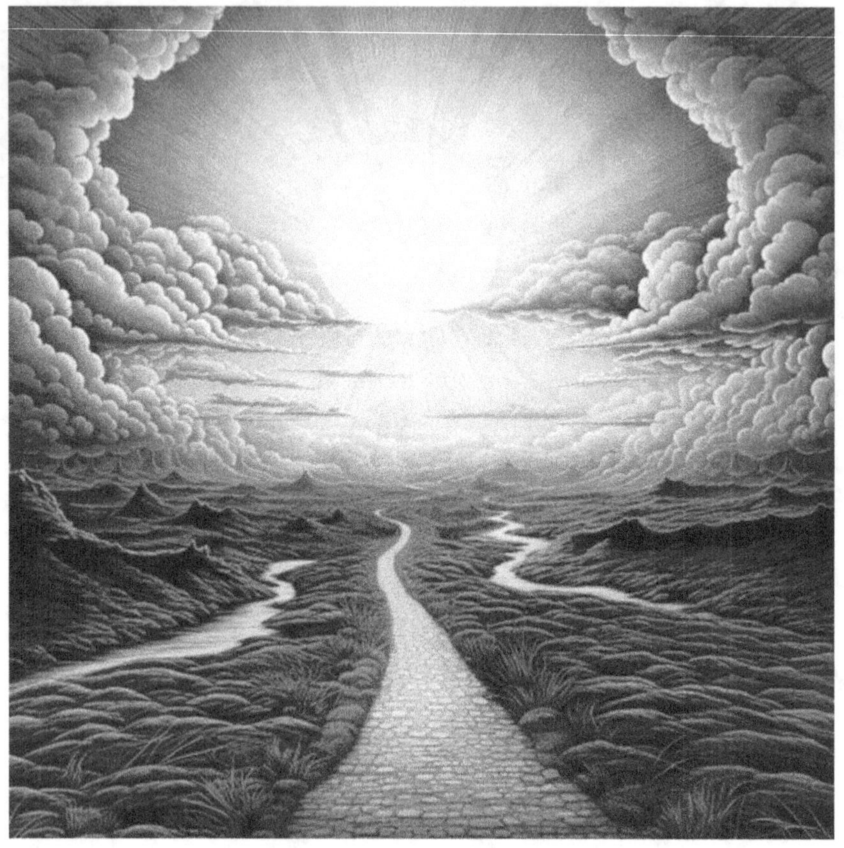

Embracing the Journey Ahead

In this remarkable journey through life's most challenging tribulations, we've discovered that the power of love, gratitude, and faith is unmatched. Every chapter of this book has been a testament to the strength of the human spirit, the unwavering love of family and friends, and the boundless grace of a higher power. The battles with cancer, the ups and downs, the moments of doubt, and the triumphant days of hope—each one was an important lesson, a stepping stone to finding true purpose and understanding.

I wish to impart to you, dear reader, that no matter the adversities you face, there lies within you an immense reservoir of strength. My journey, from the depths of despair to the peaks of gratitude, is a beacon for all who are navigating through their own challenges. Remember, life's beauty isn't just in its perfect moments, but in the resilience we display during the tough ones. The sun shines brightest after the storm.

With each sunrise comes a new opportunity, a chance to be reborn, to rediscover yourself, and to embrace the simple joys of life. Let's not search for happiness in grand milestones, but find it in the everyday moments—a kind word, a heartfelt laugh, a genuine connection.

If this book has touched your heart or provided even a glimmer of hope, I kindly ask you to share your experience. Your words could be the beacon for someone else in their time of need. Please consider leaving a review on *Amazon*, letting others know how these stories and lessons resonated with you.

As we close this chapter, always remember: *Life is a precious gift. Celebrate it, cherish it, and most importantly, live it with love, faith, and gratitude. The journey is yours to embrace, and you are never alone in it.*

Resources

American Institute for Cancer Research. (n.d.). *Blog.* https://www.aicr.o
rg/resources/blog/

Antioxidants and cancer prevention. (2017, February 6). National Cancer
Institute. https://www.cancer.gov/about-cancer/causes-prevention/
risk/diet/antioxidants-fact-sheet

Cancer Research UK. (n.d.). *Cancer Research UK.* https://www.cancerrese
archuk.org/

Cruciferous vegetables and cancer prevention. (2012, June 7). National
Cancer Institute. https://www.cancer.gov/about-cancer/causes-preve
ntion/risk/diet/cruciferous-vegetables-fact-sheet

Eating Hints: Before, during, and after Cancer Treatment. (n.d.). National
Cancer Institute. https://www.cancer.gov/publications/patient-educat
ion/eating-hints

*Information and Resources about for Cancer: Breast, Colon, Lung, Prostate,
Skin.* (n.d.). American Cancer Society. https://www.cancer.org/

Nutrition for People with Cancer | American Cancer Society. (n.d.). American
Cancer Society. https://www.cancer.org/cancer/survivorship/coping/
nutrition.html

OpenAI. (2023). ChatGPT. OpenAI. https://www.openai.com/chatgpt

Sleep Foundation. (2023, March 3). *Sleep Foundation | Better Sleep for a Better You.* https://www.sleepfoundation.org/

Top-ranked hospital in the nation – Mayo Clinic. (n.d.). Mayo Clinic. https://www.mayoclinic.org/

WCRF International. (2022, September 5). *Resources and toolkits - WCRF International.* https://www.wcrf.org/diet-activity-and-cancer/global-cancer-update-programme/resources-and-toolkits/

WCRF International. (2023, September 11). *Cancer Prevention Organisation | World Cancer Research Fund International - WCRF International.* https://www.wcrf.org/